Contents

Introduction 1

Chapter 1 3

  WHAT IS A GOOD DIET? 3

What is the Keto diet? 3

  WHY AVOID AN UNHEALTHY DIET 6

Chapter 2 9

  DIET MOTIVATION 9

  THE PSYCHOLOGY OF SELF-MOTIVATION 10

    Number 1: Can you do it? 10

    Number 2: How prepared are you? 11

    Number 3: Is it worth it? 12

    Number 4: Be accountable to someone 13

Chapter 3 14

GOAL ADVERSARIES AND HOW TO DEFEAT THEM 14

    The mind 14

    Fear 15

    Put yourself in charge 15

    Believe 15

    Rid your mind of excuses 16

Chapter 4 20

  HOW TO SET REALISTIC TARGETS 20

    Define where you are right now 20

    Determine what you want to achieve 21

    Do some research 22

    Genuine goals 24

    Flexible aims 24

    Commitment 25

    External obstacles 26

Progress stage..26

Other companions to your project...27

Chapter 5 28

THE LINK BETWEEN DIET AND PRODUCTIVITY.................................28

Do not eat junk food...28

Caffeine 29

Breakfast 29

Lunch 30

Don't forget to Hydrate...31

Chapter 6 33

HAVING A SOCIAL SUPPORT NETWORK 33

It reduces the risks of isolation..33

Social support motivates..34

YOU, YOUR DIET, AND THE MEDIA...35

Chapter 7 38

STOPPING THE UNHEALTHY DIET CRAZE 38

Eat whole and fresh foods. 40

Conclusion 43

References...45

You know what to do to lose weight.
But there is no motivation. Let's get
some motivation.

Introduction

The innumerable amount of health issues linked to problems from our diets underscores the importance of having a proper diet. We know that a bottle of soda isn't healthy, but we still gulp it. Enlightenment campaigns on the dangers of obesity have been started and concluded, but John, who lives in Denver, Colorado, will again eat that hamburger when everyone has gone to bed.

About a third of US adults are suffering from obesity, and approximately 17% of children and adolescents between the ages of 2 and 19 are obese. It is a sorry situation, especially when kids are diagnosed with illnesses that were, in times past, the exclusive reserve of adults. Children are coming down with fatty liver diseases, osteoporosis, and hypertension. Type 2 diabetes and high levels of cholesterol are now a thing in kids. It wouldn't be surprising to find a woman suffering from obesity, and her 7-year-old child has Type 2 diabetes. Our diet plays a role in the occurrence of these illnesses.

We must control what we eat. Making a list, something in the form of a schedule that details what we eat in the morning and other times in a day is an excellent start. However, this schedule, like other routines, gets monotonous. We get tired, and in a little time, we go back to the unhealthy carbs that make us bloat and ultimately achieve obesity. The solution isn't in streamlining what we take into our stomach; we need to destroy the urge for the harmful foods we take. It is essential to suppress the trigger that makes us go back to that unhealthy diet. We need to motivate ourselves to see these unhealthy diets for what they are: a danger to our health. What's more, when we fall ill because of unhealthy meals, we spend money to care for ourselves with gym memberships, drugs, etc. We must now employ concrete and decisive steps to fight an unhealthy diet and lifestyle.

In this book, we will learn about what constitutes a proper keto diet and how to stay motivated while at it. We will know how to differentiate between good and bad food. This work seeks to make clear the various steps you'll take to fight those triggers from your head. You will learn how to stay motivated as you begin your journey on the right diet plant. It will provide you intimate guidelines on what you need in your quest to lose weight. It will help you defeat that mindset that is holding you back. It is a companion you wouldn't want to be without if you're concerned about your health.

Chapter 1

WHAT IS A GOOD DIET?

We've heard several times about the importance of a proper diet to our body, and sometimes, we're left to guess what food to add and what food not to eat.

Our bodies need proper and regular nutrition from our food. A proper healthy and balanced diet should provide the body all it requires to function at an optimum level.

The Keto (Ketogenic) diet is an excellent diet that would provide our body with the right amount of nutrient. Contrary to what most people think, the ketogenic diet is not a new diet trend, neither is it a fad diet. The ketogenic diet has been scientifically studied over the years was first created for children with epilepsy because it reduced the frequency of epileptic seizures.

What is the Keto diet?

The Ketogenic diet is a low carb, high-fat diet. Therefore, the diet works by drastically cutting away carbohydrates but enriching your body with proteins and fats. It is a diet that causes the body to release ketones into the bloodstream as a reaction. When you eat foods that are low in carbohydrates, the diet pushes your body to burn fats rather than carbohydrates. Usually, the carbs will be converted to glucose and used around the body as energy. So, without that carbohydrate source, your liver will work on fat and convert it to fatty acids and ketone bodies. These ketone bodies will become the body's energy source. At that stage, when your body has elevated level of ketone bodies, this is called ketosis. There are lots of reasons why the keto diet is good. It significantly reduces glucose energy source, to drive metabolism, while making sure your body has all the nutrients you need to function optimally. The keto diet is a prime example of a proper diet because:

1. **It improves your general well-being:** When you eat healthily, you are more active, mentally, and physically. The keto diet fills your body with essential fats, vitamins, minerals, and little of carbohydrates to improve your general health. A minute amount of carbohydrate in your diet will save you from heart trouble and help to prevent weight gain.

2. **It helps you save money:** Most people are oblivious to the fact that unhealthy eating is costlier than healthy eating. In 2008, Barrack Obama's campaign was in full swing. He proposed, amongst other things, preventive medicine. Based on a post by Newsweek, $2.1 trillion was spent on healthcare in 2007 in the US, and out of this, 95 cents of every dollar spent on medical care was for treating a disease. So, instead of prevention, instead of being cautious and eating healthy, this money was spent on cures. If you are indulging in unhealthy meals, you will lose money to medical care. So, why not embrace a diet that is clean for a little extra Benjamin's? The keto diet encourages low carb food that are clean like leafy greens, fatty fish, and fresh meat. When you eliminate those bad food choices, you discover that this high quality and clean diet is the best decision for your health. That dollar you spent buying a milkshake or a hamburger might be what will cost you a thousand dollar in surgical bills. Be smart and eat wisely.

3. **It helps you maintain a healthy weight:** With a proper diet, you can maintain and manage a healthy level of weight. The keto diet can help anyone lose weight within the first few months. After losing all that extra weight, the keto diet can help sustain the weight loss for a long time. As a diet that is filled with nutritional essentials like vegetables, protein, and dairy, amongst others, the keto diet will help you place your health at a higher level.

4. **With keto, you focus better and concentrate more:** Because your body runs on keto power, it improves cognitive functions, which mean you will gain higher mental clarity and performance. On the other hand, foods that are high in cholesterol and fat can inflict significant damage in the brain by building plaques in brain vessels, causing

stroke and destroying brain tissues. When you eat the keto diet, your mind stays healthy and engaged.

5. **Improves and clears up brain fog:** The keto diet can only increase mental clarity but has been proven to help with conditions like anxiety and depression. More scientific studies also discovered that the keto diet could reverse the effects of neuron problems like Dementia, Parkinson's disease, Alzheimer's disease and possibly delay brain aging.

6. **It helps cell regeneration:** No one likes to see their face or hands wrinkled as signs of aging. Sometimes, it leads to panicky reactions like spending vast sums of money on different types of balms and lotions to fight skin aging. You can prevent wrinkles today if you make the right decisions. Dark leafy greens like kale and broccoli are excellent sources of Vitamin C. Also, avocados, berries, fish, and nuts contain vital vitamins and minerals that are essential to good skin. Vitamin C helps to construct collagen, which will make your skin firmer and reduce the rate of premature aging. Berries are good sources of vitamins and antioxidants, and eating them improves the regeneration of cells for new skin. Apart from this, you also need a diet that can improve your stomach health. Scientific studies show that the keto diet can help regenerate cells in the intestine and help us recover from damages in those areas.

7. **Keto provides sustained energy:** Foods containing high simple carbohydrates are well known for their crashes. In only a few hours after ingesting them, we may need to eat something because our body has depleted those energy sources. This makes us to feel sluggish and crave more energy in form of sugar and carbs. With the keto diet, our fat intake is the main source of energy for the day. A fatty breakfast is highly recommended. You can take four cups of keto coffee in the morning. It could be black tea or coffee with 1 tablespoon of MCT oil or ghee. You can also try mushroom coffee with any of the above fats. Give it a shot! You might like it.

8. **It reduces the incidences of chronic diseases:** Healthy diets reduce your exposure to chronic diseases. According to the Center for Disease Control (CDC), risk factors for diseases like Type 2 diabetes have been on a steady increase due to unhealthy eating habits and weight gain. Diabetes remains the leading cause of blindness and kidney failure amongst people ages 20 to 74. These diseases are a reflection of the kinds of food we eat. Those with healthy nutritional habits won't find themselves in such categories. The keto diet can help you lose fat that is connected to metabolic syndrome, prediabetes, and Type 2 diabetes. It can also help to improve sensitivity to insulin.

9. **Keto can improve our heart health**: Our heart is one of the most critical organs in the body. We must take care of it to sustain health. The keto diet can reduce blood pressures, blood sugars, LDL cholesterol levels (this is bad for your health), and body fat. With all of these out of the way, the keto can bring positive impacts on your heart because you are less likely to have high blood pressure, heart failure, hardened arteries, and other heart conditions.

WHY AVOID AN UNHEALTHY DIET

An unhealthy diet is one that doesn't give the body what it needs. An unhealthy diet may include highly processed items like snacks and fast foods that tend to be extremely low in nutrients like minerals, vitamins, and antioxidants, and high on empty calories because of the refined flour, sugar, and sodium used in making them. Vilma Andari, MS, CEO and co-founder of *Nutra Health Food*, once opined that the methods and ingredients used in preparing the food determine if the food is unhealthy or not. In her words, ***"Sodium, sugar, and trans-fat are key ingredients one should always monitor when eating out and shopping at the grocery store.*** Trans fat is a no-no for someone who wants to be healthy. Taking food that is super-high in sodium can increase your risk to cardiovascular disease, and sugar causes weight gain. The keto diet encourages the intake of unsaturated fats, and, according to a recent study, it is vital to watch your saturated fat intake.

An unhealthy diet will result in the following:

1. **Always feeling tired:** You'll lack energy all the time. It may be that you don't get enough of some essential nutrients like iron. When you're iron deficient, you can develop anemia, a situation where you don't have the requisite amount of red blood cells to pump and transfer nutrients and oxygen to other parts of the body. Note that being tired doesn't automatically translate to having a bad diet. It may be symptoms of other diseases like heart issues or a thyroid problem.

2. **Dry and brittle hair:** This is one of the most obvious signs of unhealthy eating. Iron, vitamin C, and folate are nutrients that are important for the growth and health of your hair. If you don't get these nutrients in the needed amounts, you might notice a change in your hair. Your skin may also change color. It may become pale and thin. Again, other health conditions may lead to these symptoms, such as a problem with the thyroid.

3. **Dental problems:** Your mouth is one of the first places that will show evidence of a poor and unhealthy diet. When you are vitamin C deficient, your gums may start to bleed. It may lead to infected gums. In extreme cases, it may cost you your teeth. If you use dentures or if you begin to lose teeth, consider changing your dietary pattern.

4. **Bruising easily and taking time to heal:** This is a typical effect of eating unhealthy foods. Falling from the table or bumping into something with little weight may cause you to bleed. It may be due to what you eat, that is, a diet being deficient in vitamin C, vitamin K, or protein, etc. Vitamin C aids tissues in repairing themselves, while vitamin K is an essential element in blood clotting. When you're deficient in all these, and you bruise, it may take time to heal.

5. **Slow response of your immune system:** A good and healthy diet improves our immune system. When that isn't the case, your immune system might not respond quickly and might not be as strong as it used to be to fight illness. Protein, zinc, and

vitamins C, A, and E are essential elements for a robust immune system. When they're absent or your body is deficient of these, your immune system will be weak.

The above are a few out of the numerous effects that may come because of a bad or unhealthy diet.

With a proper diet, our bodies get what is needed to function optimally. An unhealthy diet doesn't give the body what it wants. When the body doesn't understand what it requires to function optimally, a lot of negative health issues can occur.

You must have the required motivation and discipline to cut off the extra food that is adding calories to your diet. These excess calories aren't useful in any way but will contribute to making you sick and unhealthy. You need **"Diet Motivation."** It is the burning desire to eliminate foods that aren't useful to you, despite all the seeming difficulties, like addiction, media, advertising seduction, and other triggers. We will discuss this in the next chapter.

Chapter 2

DIET MOTIVATION

Motivation is the process of triggering, stimulating, and pushing people into actions that will lead them to the accomplishment of goals. So, **diet motivation** is the process people go through to keep their diet in check. It is what compels them to take sometimes painful but decisive actions that will ultimately lead to the health goals they want to achieve, be it weight loss or maintaining an optimum level of health.

For any endeavor to be successful, a lot of work must go into it. That work won't come about if the person isn't motivated. To conquer your dietary demons, you need the motivation to confront those things holding you back from ditching that cookie, chocolate, cake, etc.

Diet motivation helps you to manage your time efficiently so that you eat well and healthily even when you don't have the time to cook. When you engage the power of motivation, you will be able to stick to your diet plan, despite the obstacles and the lure to grab a bite. Diet motivation is useful because:

- **Motivation will help you achieve your goals.** It is through motivation that you stay concentrated on the task you want to attain.
- **Motivation helps you to prioritize.** When you are motivated, you know what to eat and what you shouldn't. It is easy to choose a healthy meal over a binge of junk food because you're adequately motivated to achieve your goal, and you have the discipline to prioritize this goal over any other thing.
- **Motivation is what makes you make actionable decisions.** Commitments made to lose weight or eat healthily might end up as words, but with motivation, you will put in the work.
- **Motivation will make lifestyle changes less overwhelming.** The switch from an unhealthy diet to a healthy one might be overwhelming. You're accustomed to

satisfying a craving, but you can't do that anymore because you're now a changed person. However, there are days when you might get tired and fall back to old habits. Some people give in and resign to their fates, but those who are adequately motivated know that setbacks and obstacles are an integral part of the process. Motivation helps you to rise and defeat all obstacles in your way.

- **Diet motivation keeps you focused and prevents you from derailing the course.**

THE PSYCHOLOGY OF SELF-MOTIVATION

Motivating other people is admittedly not an easy thing to do. It requires patience and sometimes a truckload of words to enable them to see things from your standpoint. Motivating yourself is a much bigger task, especially when the mission is to get you off something you've grown fond of.

The psychology of self-motivation involves empowering yourself with the tools you need to succeed in a goal or mission. It requires working your way up from empowerment to competence and matching it with actions. Empowering yourself is the first step to success is self-motivation. It is like a kid who wants to grow into an auto mechanic. When the dad puts him through all the required training and education, the child feels empowered to take on auto repair tasks because he has the required skills. From that point, he can motivate himself to reach higher work goals. It is the same as any other thing. To help yourself eat better, to wean yourself off those empty calories, you need to empower yourself. The keto diet you are about to embark on requires that you provide honest answers to these crucial questions. These answers should reflect your current reality. Anything other than that will jeopardize your mission before it starts.

Number 1: Can you do it?

Before you answer this, ensure that you already have the idea of what you're going to face as you embark on your journey to lose weight or eat healthily. Take a mental note of all the obstacles you're bound to face. Are you prepared for all the eventualities? Your new diet requires you to move away from your old one gradually. You need to find a way of detaching yourself from your previous unhealthy food. Now, pick a journal and document those mental notes, the obstacles, and the solutions you feel can work for you.

Outline the affirmations about the things you must let go of and how you intend to let them go. The journey you are about to embark on requires courage, patience, motivation, and discipline to attain this level of empowerment. But ultimately, it requires a full awareness of the next few months. When you write down all the areas you believe you might have limitations, it helps prepare you to overcome them.

Secondly, the reason we are talking about a written plan is that a mental note or merely visualizing where you want to be is not enough. Write down every detail about the lifestyle you already live and the areas you must work on to transform and sustain you as you embark on this fantastic journey. This exercise is the "training" and "education" you need to feel empowered. Again, you must stay honest to yourself and provide answers that will aid you in tackling the issue head-on.

Number 2: How prepared are you?

The second question is one that mirrors your preparedness more than anything. Because you have chosen the keto diet, you need to define your strategy to use it.

- What food recipes would you have?
- How would you structure your food budget to take the hit?
- Will you cook at weekends to make sure you resist temptation?
- How is your professional life?
- Should you subscribe to a keto snack plan or prepare your snacks ahead?
- How should you avoid using the snack stash at the office?
- Do you work at home? Would it be better to eliminate all those unhealthy choices from your home altogether?
- Should you eat more at home than in restaurants? What can you get from the food vendor down the street that is keto-friendly?

Understanding the different scenarios that surround your life will help you make sure the new diet plan works. When you think about your favorite restaurants and local diners, you can create a layout about the things you can eat there that are keto-friendly. If you should avoid those areas for the next few months, you can also draw a set plan in that direction. Set targets about how you far you will go with the keto diet and what you will do as you gradually get into ketosis. When you set realistic goals and make the right preparations, you can get to your destination in no time. You have to acknowledge that the change you seek is not going to come suddenly. It is going to be a gradual process, so you need to go easy on yourself. Don't set your keto plan so rigid that you immediately want to relapse to your old habit of hoarding yogurts, cakes, and cookies in your stomach sometime past 2 a.m. Because you are using the keto diet, you won't sacrifice so much. The keto plan has a lot of healthy and delicious options. You can enjoy keto pizzas, bread, muffins, and even keto lasagnas.

It is helpful to compare your notes with others. These patterns you've set, how do they compare with others who have gone the same route and have ended with the results you seek? The answer will make it easy for you to make any adjustment.

When you're satisfied that everything has been taken care of and you are convinced that this method you've employed won't be too hard on you but will still lead you to the same results, you're now empowered and competent. Your self-motivation exercise machine is up and running. The next question prepares you for the job.

Number 3: Is it worth it?

Create a list of the reasons why you are sticking to these healthy food choices. This list will shadow your goals. Is this change from eating unhealthy to healthy eating worth it? Will the risks and pains you had to endure at this stage be worth it at the end? Will you prefer to eat well and have good skin while you age or prefer to stomach all the junk and fast food and watch your skin lose its essence as you age? Do you want to avoid diabetes or conquer it? Would you love to stop having a hard time walking around your neighborhood? Do you want to be faster, agile, and less prone to illness? Would you like to develop lean muscles? Write that list and make it handy. You can also set it on reminder, so you can always remember the things that made you go on this journey. It will help you stay on track. These questions link to the first big question. The purpose of motivating yourself to eat healthily is so that you can have a healthy life. Your body can get what it needs to function effectively. With this end goal in mind, will you be ready to sacrifice your money, time, and effort to ensure that you fulfill your objective?

The position of this last question concerning the others is poignant because it assumes that you are empowered after answering the first question. It assumes that you are competent, and after providing an answer to the second question, it implies that you're aware of the intricacies of the entire process. After preparing you for everything, it concludes by asking you to weigh your options and this time, your eating habits. Will eating healthy help you in the long run? Of course, it will. Will weaning yourself off unhealthy eating habits be an easy task? Of course not, but will it be worth it? Will it be worth it avoiding those craving when you pass by a cake vendor? Yes, it will!

You are responsible for all the answers to these questions. You are building your psyche to withstand the rigors of the process. You are stimulating yourself into taking decisive action. You are motivating yourself!

Number 4: Be accountable to someone

To avoid skipping on your plan, you can let a friend or partner in on your new diet plan. On our own, it can be challenging to go on, especially on days when we feel as though we have taken a ridiculous step. This friend or partner will not bug you about losing weight, but they will encourage you, so you don't feel alone on this incredible journey. When you feel obliged to another person, it will reinforce your commitment to the end goal. It is encouraging to have someone saying "You can do it" when we are right in the middle of our great journey, sometimes, it's just about hearing that for us to finish out strong.

Chapter 3

GOAL ADVERSARIES AND HOW TO DEFEAT THEM

Healthy eating is quite hard for those who are accustomed to eating fast food. The shift to healthy diet might not be prepared for, and as such, they fall back to old habits after making commitments to eating healthy. They get pulled back by old habits and rather than identifying such tendencies and fighting them to a standstill. They succumb to the lure of the taste of the icing that adorns the top of their favorite cake and that crunchy pepperoni that sits pretty atop a slice of their favorite pizza brand. Here, we'll learn what these obstacles are and develop ways of defeating all of them.

The mind

Obstacles to your diet goals are numerous, and they start with your mind. Your mind is the most potent part of your body, the epicenter. It is the place that keeps other body parts trudging on the path to achieving your diet goals. When the mind isn't fired up enough or doesn't see the need to go through the work of leaving your favorite indulgences, your diet war will suffer, and you might not make any progress at all.

You need to program your mind to stay aligned with your diet goals. To achieve this, you need to break your goals into blocks. When you cut them into chunks, it becomes easy to follow what you are doing and find focus.

Get the journal you have been keeping as discussed in the previous chapter. Write down the little healthy habits that will transform your diet and lifestyle. Visualize how the day after today would look. What are your plans for that day? How can you fit into your new-found journey? Visualize all the crucial things you can do to make it work. What time do you go to bed? Should you sleep earlier to make time to prepare meals in the morning? For some people, working at night is typical. Should you cook at weekends? If you have to snack when working at night, what keto choices can be used? Visualize all of these and write them down. According to science, it takes 21 days of constant practice to form a habit. So, write your 21 days diet goals in the journal and aim to accomplish it so you can be healthy, have the weight you want, and save your money from illnesses.

Fear

When you're done prepping your mind, you already have enough motivation to last you through your journey. The next step is to conquer your fears. You won't do that by not admitting them and running away from them. You overcome your fears by confronting and defeating them. Usually, you'll feel nervous because you're about to change a thing or two about your life. Whether you aim for a healthy body or weight loss, the keto diet is the surefire way to accomplish your diet goals. You won't be giving up your cookies or desserts because the keto diet has great variants that are yummy. Avoid telling yourself that you are not ready to take on that change. We often have fears because we set rigid plans for ourselves and develop the "all or nothing" approach. You don't need to save up money to afford a fantastic keto plan or get a personal trainer. Start with something that works for you and build as you go on. As I said in the previous section, create your 21 days diet plan. This plan gives you something to work towards for a healthier personality.

Whenever you can resist the temptation to indulge in unhealthy food as you proceed on this journey, your plan stays intact. You are a long way out of the old lifestyle. A slight deviation won't matter in the long run.

Put yourself in charge

After acknowledging what needs to be changed, you must believe that you are the one to spearhead that change. The responsibility falls solely on your shoulder, and there is no chance of delegation. You're the one to make the decisions. You're the one who will ensure that the plans you've outlined are followed. It is your dance, and you should dictate the music you want.

Believe

The last step is to believe that you can do it. You need to affirm your ability to bring about that change you desire. Your failures in the past shouldn't get in the way of your present efforts. You must believe that you're up to the task and take the necessary actions to back up that belief.

Rid your mind of excuses

Tell yourself that reasons to relapse no longer hold water. Don't allow any justification to get in your way of living a healthy life. Don't excuse yourself from responsibilities. Weigh the advantages of living and eating healthily compared to the dangers of eating unhealthy foods and being overweight. Use this to motivate yourself not to give in to excuses. In life, flimsy reasons will stop you from getting results, but actions and responsibilities will provide you with results.

You have to fire your mind up into being committed to the entire process. You can't claim to want to lose weight and go about eating everything you want because you plan to do intermittent fasting for a day or two. That is self-sabotage. The gap between success and failure is occupied by commitment. It can swing the results both ways. Give your exercise or your proper diet the same priority and importance as you do to other things in your life. If you put in work, you'll see results, but if you don't, nothing will come out of the process.

Now that your mind is charged, you're ready to take on other obstacles, including:

1. **Setting realistic goals:** In your admirable desire to hit the ground running and achieve as much as possible in record time, do not set goals that are at parallels with reality. We often look for the perfect keto plan, the ideal exercise plan, or even the perfect environment. There is no such thing as losing weight right now. There is no such thing as switching from unhealthy to healthy eating in one fell swoop. But you can reach your targets when your goals talk about what you can do in the next hour or two. Let your goals work with your plans for tonight. What can you prepare for your family? Will you have deserts as well? Are you going to see a friend? What can you eat there? Realistic plans are concrete, measurable and timely. For instance, in the long term, you could aim to lose about 500-700 calories daily and it is healthy too. One kilogram of body weight is about 7,777 calories. This means that having a calorie deficit of about 700 calories daily will cause 1 kg weight loss in 10 days. The keto diet is helpful because it uses up fat rather than glucose in a high-carb diet.

Also, it is a great idea to set diet plans based on the real-time you have lunch or dinner or the mid-day snack you love having. This will work for you. You need to understand that it is a gradual process. When you set realistic goals, have fun in the process.

2. **Short-term change:** Imagine that you've endured the process and done all the right things. Your body has adjusted and responded accordingly. After you've hit the goal you had in mind, you start to relax and end up quitting. Weight begins to pile up, your body becomes susceptible to illness, and you have to start everything over. When you commit to the keto diet, you need to understand that it is a lifetime process. Therefore, whatever you do now will change your lifestyle forever. You shouldn't pause or stop the process when you've achieved your aim. You must make adjustments to accommodate the life changes needed to sustain the goals you've achieved. Keto provides avenues to alternate between the full meal plan and the keto plan after you have reached your optimal weight loss goal. It is one of the reasons why the keto diet is better than crash diets. You can sustain it throughout your life without sacrificing anything.

3. **"Exercise eating":** Does this sound familiar? Yes! Some people exercise or go to the gym and when they're done sweating out the excess calories; these people believe that they have the dieting freedom to eat whatever they want. They think that their workout will cancel out what they've just eaten. This is a wrong notion. At times, not going to the gym is better than going there and stuffing your stomach with food you're trying to avoid. When you do this, what you've eaten hasn't settled in your body and what you've sweated out has nothing to do with what you've just eaten. While exercise is essential, your diet is as crucial. Visiting the gym might not shield your body from the effects of eating unhealthily.

4. **Commitment:** You've made a visual representation of how you want your body to be and have started making all the right decisions to ensure that you hit that point. You've fallen a few times, but this time is different. You're determined, and you want to see this through. After a few weeks of doing the right thing, you started getting sloppy. At

first, it started as simple as eating some cake when everyone else went to bed. You assured yourself that you could do it and told yourself not to bother because it wouldn't happen again. But it did happen again. You're getting weak, and slowly, your focus erodes. You are finding excuses when there aren't any to skip gym sessions. You think you deserve a bag of popcorn and a can of soda because you've done an excellent job in the past weeks. Before you know it, you're back at ground zero, where everything started. The efforts you put in will amount to nothing. This is one of the reasons why we must create that plan for the first two weeks and adjust accordingly by the end of the first two weeks to work for the next two weeks. A lot of experts recommend writing goals up to 21 days, but a lot of people have a lot of events happening around them that might thwart those plans for 21 days long. Holding on for 14 days and then pushing for the next 14 days is worth it. There's nothing more exciting than the drive to attain a goal because it is only a few days longer.

Before you made this commitment, it might have been reasonable for you to wake up at 2 a.m. and walk to your fridge to have a bite of the chocolate velvet cake you kept for breakfast. That is reasonable because you were hungry. But now you're supposed to eat healthily. You're limited to a certain number of calories you can consume daily. Some people can't survive the lure of satisfying their hunger with their favorite junk food.

The process takes a lot from you, but you have to look at the bigger picture. You need to get healthy. Eat healthy so that your body gets what it requires to function optimally.

Unhealthy diets might cost less in the front. However, they will give you a great economic loss due to medication and all other adverse side effects in the long run. Unhealthy diets will continuously weaken the body until it can't bear it anymore. It is akin to paying to make you sick. In as much as a healthy diet may hit your pocket, it shouldn't be an excuse for you to eat unhealthily and moreover, you'll be getting more than enough value for your money. You will live out your young age in health, and as you age, rather than having a wrinkling skin, yours will glow, all thanks to the sacrifices you made while you were younger.

Don't allow the fear of paying a few extra bucks to push you into eating unhealthy foods. It's better, safer, and healthier! Also, there are cheaper alternatives.

Remember that it all rests on you. Fight it! Don't lose!

Chapter 4

HOW TO SET REALISTIC TARGETS

As it is with everything that involves planning and getting results, there is a need to set targets that are not only realistic but achievable. The following tips will help you in that course.

Define where you are right now

Motivating yourself into eating healthy is great, but you have to determine your current situation. You have to go through the required tests to see the extent of the damage, if there is any, that unhealthy diet has caused to your body. Look at external sources if there is a need. When you are fully aware of your present situation, you will be very clear on the work that needs to be done. It will be another method of motivating yourself because you might not like what you see. It will increase your commitment to the course and help you as you make food eating and dietary decisions. Any decision you make will be built on what you know. With this, you'll hit the ground running. So, let's get started, pick up that journal and start documenting:

- How much do you weigh?
- Describe your family goals
- Describe your professional situation
- What kind of financial plan do you have in place? How will it define your diet plan?
- Are you responsible for other people not directly related to you?
- What is your health situation? How would the keto plan work around it?
- Are you breastfeeding? Or do you have kids whose means will contradict with your own? Is there a way to bring them to love keto so your family will remain united?
- Do you spend more time on your feet or off it? Is your current energy intake too much or too little for what you do?

- Will you have time to cook your meals? Or are you better off, subscribing to a local place that can make those keto meals for you?
- Should you cook alone or pair up with a close friend, so it's easier to watch what you eat?

Determine what you want to achieve

You might want to lose weight or gain a better immune system, clear skin, or sharp eyes; those are all general goal plans. Here, I want you to write what you want to achieve in two weeks. According to Dr. Mark Hyman, the only way to make the next two weeks work for you is by focusing on the process and not the outcome. Don't set the amount of weight you want to lose. Most people will have inconsistent weight that will go higher a bit and then come back down after a while. Not everyone can watch their weight which they already feel is too high and feel good about it. Instead of focusing on the weight you want to achieve, set goals like this:

- I want my weekend with friends to be keto packed, so I am going to have X food or Y drink
- I will love a midnight snack on Wednesday while I work, so a few nuts, an avocado slice or a cup of tea should do the trick
- I want to begin my day with sunshine, so I would love that keto coffee for breakfast before I work, and by noon, I have this keto meal for brunch.
- Should I bring in Intermittent fasting to save a few extra dollars to spend on Y keto lunch and dinner?
- Will my parents visit in a few hours? Should I cook some special keto meal we can all enjoy or take them out, so it's not too restrictive for them?

These are all realistic goals because they focus on what is going on in your life. They provide a clear picture of what will happen in a few hours. So, tailor your goals to match those hours. Never generalize because you are unique and fantastic. You have lots of commitments besides your meals. Make sure you write those details down, so it becomes easier to follow them. Structure them to fit by the hour and minute. When you have a detailed outlook of what you want to achieve, it guides you to the path you have chosen whenever you are tempted to lose track.

Do some research

The importance of being informed cannot be overstated. You need as much information as you can get. It may be the first time you hear about calories or how eating unhealthily might weaken your body's ability to protect itself.

You need the information to know the number of calories food X and food Y has respectively. Most people don't even know how much calories an apple has. But they have eaten an apple 100 of times in their life. Does it have 40, 100 or 150 calories?

Information is the only way you know the effects of consistently consuming food Z. Knowing what other people have experienced in their journey to healthy eating will also help. How much will your diet cost you? What part of your lifestyle triggers you into consuming unhealthy foods? How long will it take before the change you seek starts to appear? You will be in a better position to tackle any of the above issues and more because you have done your research. Not being educated about nutrition is like driving through the city without knowing what the traffic signs mean. It's dangerous. Suicide might look too hard, but the message here is that research can save you a lot of trouble.

Don't go blindly into changing your diet. Be informed and know what you're doing. Ask questions on gray areas and immediately seek the help of a professional when problematic symptoms emerge.

Tip: A few insights on keto calories

The calories we eat in our food are what gives our bodies the energy to function. Calories are what our bodies use to power walking, thinking, breathing, and other essential body works.

On average, our bodies need about 2,000 calories daily to sustain their present weight level. Individual differences like gender, age, and physical activity levels may bring about differences. Naturally, men need more calories than women, and those who engage in physical activities that demand lots of energy need more. The United States Department of Agriculture (USDA) <u>guidelines</u> gave examples of daily calories intake. It stated that for kids between the ages of 2 to 8, their regular consumption should be between 1,000–1,400 calories. Girls between the ages of 9 to 13 should consume between 1,400 to 1,600 calories. Boys in the same age range should consume 1,600 to 2,000 calories daily. Active women between the ages 14 and 30 should up their consumption to 2,400 calories if they're consuming lower than that. Sedentary women within that age range should consume between 1,800–2,000 calories. Active men within the 14 to 30 age range should consume between 2,800 and 3,000 calories. Sedentary men within that age range should have 2,000 to 2,600 calories. Active men and women who are more than 30 years of age should consume 2,000 to 3,000 calories, and sedentary women and men who are more than 30 years of age should consume between 1,600 to 2,400 calories.

Not all calories are excellent and the same as most people think. This is mainly due to differences in the source of the food. Some calories are called "empty calories" because they add little or no nutritional value to the body. The USDA defines "empty calories" as calories from solid fats like butter and sugar. It is important to note that all butters aren't the same. The keto diet encourages the intake of natural grass-fed butter. According to the USDA, most Americans fill their body with these empty calories when they consume ice cream, cookies, pizza, energy drinks, fruit drinks, cakes, sausages, sports drinks, and soda. In other words, we are surrounded by things that are of no value to our health, but we keep consuming them with a constant frequency. This goes a long way to reinforce the point that you need discipline and motivation to dump these bad habits for good habit and a proper diet.

However, what you find here is only general information. On the keto diet, you will receive much lower calories than the recommended. Your keto food choices can determine those calories for you because a lot of keto recipes are already created, bearing in mind the calorie content that would work. So, check out the necessary information on ketogenic diet needs and how to mix recipes to stay on the keto side. You don't have to count calories obsessively, but learning will help you strategize properly.

Genuine goals

Now armed with information, your goals shouldn't only be a reflection of your values, but they should also be practical. They should be things you know you can do. Don't compare yourself with others because every individual is different. What worked for that person might not work for you, and what works for you might not work for the other. This doesn't preclude you from looking to them for guidance. You can set tasks for yourself that is a bit challenging and maybe even a bit of a stretch, but they shouldn't be hopeless so that failure to achieve those goals will be demoralizing. In deciding what you seek to achieve, you must answer these questions: Why should I give up unhealthy eating? Is it worth it? Why should I give up everything sweet because I want to eat healthily?

Flexible aims

The goals you've set, apart from being realistic, should be manageable, measurable, and fun. There should be space for your goals to accommodate recent and relevant discoveries. Life isn't static, and because we're living in it, we will see new things that are better than what we know. Your plan should create allowances for little alterations for the greater good.

Also, your goals shouldn't be vague. Make your goals in such a way that you can monitor your progress and note your lapses. At the end of your day, write down what you did about your diet. Did you drink water three times? How many liters? Did you have a little bread along the way? Did you have a hard time preparing your lunch or dinner? Was breakfast at the time you planned? Did your kids love the keto plan you developed? Is there a way to make them love it? When you write everything you did for that day, you can make adjustments for the next day. Maybe you need to drink more water at the start of the day. You might need to stop thinking about preparing your lunch since it makes you late to work, maybe you need to check out some local diners that can deliver a modified keto lunch to your office. Your friend might be hosting a birthday bash, tomorrow night, so, you should probably inform them about your meal choices and eat something earlier than necessary to make sure you are too full to dive into the temptations that might arise at that party.

You know that you have to keep the fire burning if you're making progress or that you have to step up if you aren't. With measurable plans, you know exactly how far you've come in achieving your target. It is another form of motivation because looking back and seeing the efforts you've put in will no doubt spur you into doing more. It can also come in handy when you want to give up. Never fail to write down everything you do at the end of the day. When you write and review, it will be easier to make sure that the next day accommodates those circumstances.

Your target shouldn't be some rehashed academic one-liner. Make it fun. It should be something you enjoy doing. Don't make it too hard on yourself such that you're looking to stop as quickly as you started. Be innovative. Understand that it is your life, so make it fun, colorful, and enjoyable.

Commitment

Commitment to the course is the fuel you need to stay in line throughout the journey. With dedication, you won't waver in the face of difficulty. As you're making plans, you must gauge the level of involvement you have. Unhealthy eating might be something you are used to. It may be such that you've developed a sort of craving for it so leaving it in the past will not be easy. You need to ask yourself and provide yourself with the answers you need to gauge your commitment level. Are you ready to see it through? Are you committed to ensuring that you give it your best shot? These questions and more will help you.

Another issue that may reduce or tamper with your level of commitment is your limitations. Limitations come in different forms. For example, now that you're eating healthy, your pocket may be taking a hit. There are healthy, cheaper alternatives. Or maybe you work in a pizza factory, and the lure of your favorite food pointing at you is too hard to resist. If you consider the economic loss to medications, imagine your weight bloated, think about yourself in the gym trying to cut down the weight you could prevent in the first place, you will agree that a healthy diet is much more important than holding to such job. Even when a job switch sounds exhausting, it's necessary if it will affect your health positively. What is more, it's also a great commitment.

External obstacles

External obstacles that will hinder you are innumerable. One example is being friends with people who like to go on a sugary diet consumption binge. When these kinds of triggers surround you, your journey will be fraught with problems. Just like your limitations, you have to own up to your external obstacles and tackle them. Methods of defeating them are solely on you, and that can be difficult.

What you should do is surround yourself with people that will help you with your new plans. You don't have to cut people from your life. You can bring one special friend close to you, who will understand your unique goals and encourage you on that path. If you can't fight anyone around you who would appreciate those goals, get a new friend. There are lots of people who are also on this journey with you. You can meet them at the local health club, the fitness unit or even online. Make commitments with them, and you can push each other to succeed. Working in pairs or groups brings a lot of unity because you all share the same ultimate goal. Get on your feet and look for that special friend or partner you can be accountable to. If you can't find one in your immediate circle, go out and look for a new friend.

Progress stage

You've made progress. Everything looks good. You're visualizing yourself in that body you've always dreamed of, courtesy of these newly found healthy eating habits. You might want to pause to revise everything you've planned. When you review and change, it will make you see problems with your plans, if any. Moreover, going over your plan again is another way of ensuring that you've captured everything you want. It gives you the chance to add or subtract from the plan.

If you're sure that everything is in order, then wait no further! Get to work! Follow your plan meticulously and don't act outside of it. Don't give room for the slightest of excuses. Your eyes should fixate on your target so that no obstacle will make you consider quitting. Put in time and effort! Remind yourself of the reasons that pushed you in the first place.

Your body will thank you in a short while! Once you've gotten into the thick of the action, make sure you track your progress. Keep records.

With the above, your target just got a lot easier. You can personalize your plan to fit your peculiarities.

Other companions to your project

The first is a mechanism that helps you fight against all the factors that will lure you into giving up. It should be a mechanism that insulates you from the plethora of temptations you'll encounter along the way. You can decide to start with your mind. You may choose to cut eating ties with members of your clique who suffer from the same problem.

Your defense mechanism should make space for potential setbacks. If it couldn't stop you from caving into having a bite on Monday, it should prevent you from eating unhealthy foods every other day of the week. Make sure that the mechanism is efficient to prevent you from caving into having another bite.

The next one is celebrating yourself. When you hit a certain level of achievement after every phase, make it a point to reward your hard work. Some might say it isn't a big deal, but it is. Reward yourself with a healthy food treat — that way you give yourself something to look forward to.

However, celebrating yourself doesn't mean giving yourself a pass to eat unhealthy food for a day. You will be jeopardizing your work because eating it today means you may have reawakened your cravings. This may mean you lose everything because you have to start again. Nevertheless, if you fall off track, get up and push forward. You are a long way from where you were before, and that's enough to say that you are doing great.

Chapter 5

THE LINK BETWEEN DIET AND PRODUCTIVITY

You must have stumbled upon the age-old saying, *"you are what you eat."* It is a fact that is more pronounced when you link it to your behavior in the workplace. *"You are what you eat"* can be reworked into *"you work the way you eat."* Your diet has a significant impact on the results you produce or wish to churn out in your place of work. It is common knowledge that the human body gets energy from food consumed. The body is left with energy to function with after the digestive system uses part of that energy to digest the food. Invariably, it means that if you consume foods that don't give the body the amount of energy needed for the kind of output you want, you won't get the output you need. You must pay close attention to what you take into your body. The following are crucial but straightforward healthy eating habits that will help increase your productivity. Following these will ensure that your eyes don't get blurry three hours into a Monday morning and you won't start to wish you were a sorcerer so you can make the weekends come faster.

Do not eat junk food

This is the most common of all unhealthy foods. It is so because there are hundreds of junk foods all around us. They are highly processed snacks that contain an enormous number of calories that most times take the form of sugar and trans-fat and have almost no vitamin, fiber, or mineral content. Fitting examples include candy, soda, chips, pastries, cake, and doughnuts. Some junk foods might not be as easily recognizable as others. They are often sold in pristine marketing disguises that will coax anyone who isn't paying attention to trying it. Take fruit drinks as a good example. They have the same quantity of sugar and calories as soda. Breakfast bars are purported by manufacturers to be filled with heart-healthy whole grains. But they contain the same amount of added sugar as a candy bar, if not more. Apart from being associated with obesity, heart diseases, Type 2 diabetes, and other chronic diseases, junk foods are known to make people have a sluggish feeling because of their high trans-fat content. You're likely to experience a burst of energy and a quick crash after eating junk foods because of the high sugar content. When any of the above happens, you can't work effectively. Sluggishness isn't accepted in any working environment in any part of the world. Crashing after a burst of energy is one way of ensuring that you won't meet your daily or monthly target. You become less productive in every way, so eat healthily.

Caffeine

Caffeine is known for its ability to kick you. It doesn't supply the body with any calories per se but provides your brain with a mild stimulant that alerts it. Logically, when you started feeling tired after eating lunch with still three more hours to go, you reach for espresso or some chocolate-covered coffee beans. You're likely to experience a surge in your energy. It is advised that you watch the amount of caffeine you consume because ingesting massive amounts of caffeine into the body might give you what you want, a surge in your energy levels, but with a guaranteed crash to follow. To be and stay productive throughout the day, take only small amounts of caffeine.

Breakfast

It is not healthy to skip breakfast. As someone on the keto diet, you should know that fats compose about 70% of your keto meal. The body uses the fats to generate energy for the day rather than glucose which can pose a threat to a healthy heart and bring a myriad of health issues. The absence of glucose will deplete the glycogen stores in the body. Once these stores are depleted, the fats are used for energy and you can lose weight easily and maintain a healthy outlook.

So, for the standard keto diet plan, you must have breakfast at the start of the day. Here are some quick examples of a keto breakfast delight that should sustain you until your next meal;

- A breakfast of eggs smoked salmon or avocado.
- Bacon and Eggs
- Bacon, poached eggs and avocado
- Boiled eggs and mayonnaise with asparagus

- Keto mushroom omelet

- Keto pancakes (almond flour) and berries

When you eat this healthy, high –fat meal, you will feel full for more extended periods of the day. They also work as small meals which can boost your productivity and avoid getting a sluggish feeling as you handle the day. When you create a consistent schedule on how fuel is supplied to your body with these keto meals, your energy levels won't fluctuate indiscriminately, giving your body the chance to remain as energized as possible.

Lunch

Our eating patterns are sometimes heavily influenced by cultures and traditions. In some cultures, eating heavy for lunch is the way to go. Eating heavy may be the prescribed way of having lunch, but is it healthy for you? Will it hamper your productivity at work?

To stay focused and productive, you need to keep your lunch moderate. Eat small portions. When you eat heavy, you're likely to fall asleep. The boss walking in on you sleeping with your head on some files isn't what you want. Think about how you work during the day and plan your lunch realistically. Would you take breaks when others do, or might be stuck with some more work? Consider some keto snacks that can fit in here. Can you eat in your office or would you instead step out? Consider your options carefully because you might consider having your meal at the Café downstairs or bring something from home. Your lunch should have a good keto mix.

Make sure your lunch is enriched with oil and fat sources. These sources should include extra omega-3s. Omega-3s are essential fatty acids that are found in different nuts, oils, and fatty fishes. A lot of scientific research has been conducted to discover the benefits they can bring to the body. Studies show that omega-3s can help you fight depression and anxiety. They can help improve the health of your eyes. Omega-3s are useful for babies because they can improve brain health while they are still in the womb and when they are still early into growth. Omega-3s can be your soldiers as you battle to defeat inflammation and autoimmune diseases. For women, they can help reduce menstrual pains. When you have fat in your liver, and you want to cut it, consider the omega-3 as an option. Your bone and joint health can also improve with the aid of omega-3s.

Two types of omega-3 fatty acids, eicosapentaenoic acid (EPA) and docosahexaenoic acid (DHA) are almost exclusively found in fish oil or fatty fish. These acids are plenty in brain cells and are very active in the preservation of the cell membrane's health. Not only that, these fatty acids ensure and facilitates communication between the cells of the brain. A study was referenced in this article wherein animals were fed diets that didn't contain any omega-3 content. It led to the reduction in the amount of DHA in the brain, and deficits in memory and learning. A study conducted in 2012 by Dr. Z. S. Tan and other authors titled "Red blood cell omega-3 fatty acid levels and markers of accelerated brain damage" showed that adults who are older with lower levels of DHA had reduced brain size, a symptom of accelerated brain aging. Omega-3s are crucial for your brain to maintain its function throughout your life. When you take omega-3s, you're invariably increasing your brain's health, and at work, a healthy mind is your best companion.

You can consider nuts, cheese, berries, cucumbers, almonds, and eggs. Here are a few ideas of what would work for your keto meal plan.

- Zoodles and meatballs
- Chicken sausage
- Smoked salmon and cream cheese roll-ups
- Bacon chips
- Tuna salad
- Keto Shrimp and cauliflower rice salad
- Avocado and egg salad.

Don't forget to Hydrate

Hydration is also important. Do you know that water makes up 60% of your body? Water promotes the health of your cardiovascular organs. When you're dehydrated, your blood volume reduces. This makes your heart work harder to pump the reduced amount of blood in your body to pass oxygen to cells. This can make normal activities like walking up the stairs challenging. You can't be productive in such a state. Water is what cleans your body of toxins. Kidneys need the help of water in discharging this duty. When your body is hydrated, you may be protecting yourself from kidney stones and infections to the urinary tract. When you're hydrated, your joints and muscles work better. With hydration, the water that stays inside and outside the cells of contracting muscles provides the required nutrients and helps you to excrete waste in better ways, helping you to perform even better. This is so for those who have physical jobs. Water also helps to lubricate the joints, helping you to move around quickly. For those whose jobs entail something like this, this is one sure way of increasing productivity.

It's normal for some people to enjoy alcohol after a tough day at work. They pour themselves cup after cup, slowly drinking themselves away to sleep. While this may be good initially, because it helps them fall asleep, it may not be worth it in the long run because the effects may wear off at night or very early in the morning. Don't drink yourself to sleep if you want to be productive at work the next day.

As stated above, these are simple but essential tips that link what you eat to your output at work. Following the above tips will no doubt maintain your level of productivity at the practical level it currently is or help to improve it. It is certain that with a healthy diet, everything will go well.

Chapter 6

HAVING A SOCIAL SUPPORT NETWORK

A social support network is made up of your peers, friends, and family who share your beliefs or have acknowledged your trust in specific topics and have come together to support themselves or you as the case may be. A social support network is critical because it helps you align with people going through similar tough challenges or changes in their lives.

If you want to change from an old and unhealthy diet to eating new and healthy food, identifying triggers that make you stumble on the path to achieving your goals is essential. One of such triggers is being in the company of those who eat junk food. When you are a part of a network, and you want to quit a trait that is a signature of that network, it is only logical that you get another network that has the same aim as yours or is ready to help your quest. Staying in the same circles you were in before will no doubt hinder your success, and even if it doesn't stop it, the rate of progress you'll get is likely to be slower.

A social support network doesn't always have to be formal. It could be as simple as visiting a friend or family member and discussing ways of being attached to healthy eating. You can also find social support network on Facebook. Just head to the search bar and type keto or ketogenic groups. This is an example of one of such groups with great pictures to show how the keto diet helps - https://www.facebook.com/ketogenic/

A social support network for healthy eating is important because of the following:

It reduces the risks of isolation

Some have become so addicted to unhealthy food that the thought of leaving it for something new is enough to stir up anxiety. They are frightened by the idea of not having food as frequently as they want. When they're alone, left to face the battle themselves, everything becomes worse. Withdrawing from addiction is a delicate issue that needs all the help one can get, and this is what social support networks provide. Being part of a like-minded group, you will meet people who share the same problems as you and you can support each other. Difficulties are better faced with the company, and that is what support networks provide. You get to hear tips and valuable insights on how to defeat your challenges, making the entire process a bit easier.

Besides, the switch to healthy eating may cause emotional distress and restlessness. These are common signs of addiction withdrawal. With the support you get from a social support system, you are able to scale them quickly and successfully.

It is noteworthy that one of the reasons why some people quit their switch from an unhealthy diet to a healthy diet midway is because they had no support system or network. There was nobody to keep edging them on in moments of emotional distress and restlessness, so they fell back to unhealthy habits. This underlines the importance of a social support network.

Furthermore, addiction to unhealthy meals may cause a person to hide and feel shame, bringing about low self-esteem. It may be that a man in his late thirties is addicted to candy bars that are thought to be consumed by kids in their formative years of development. This kind of addiction may bring shame to the man and consequently, low self-esteem. The help provided by his social support network will walk him through these feelings.

Social support motivates

You are challenged to do better when you see the efforts of other people who want the same thing you do. You'll want to push yourself if you realize how far you are behind other people's progress. This is the right way of comparing efforts with other people who want the same results. Since you're aiming for the same results, it won't hurt to compare notes!

With social support networks, the quest to eat healthily can be converted to a competition of sort where people score points for doing things at the good side of the divide. It makes the entire process fun and enjoyable. It is almost impossible to derail from the original plan when you have a strong and functional social support network.

A social support system helps you to switch to a healthy lifestyle and helps you maintain that change. Others can provide information that will come in handy.

However, the bulk of whatever success you'll have in a social support group depends on you. So, stay strong!

YOU, YOUR DIET, AND THE MEDIA

The media is an essential tool of the junk food market. Beautiful pictures of hamburgers taken in serene and picture-friendly backgrounds may be endorsed by our favorite celebrity who appeared in a video or two taking a bite. There could also be a hashtag challenge of a one-minute video of you eating a particular brand of pizza or a war of words and emotions on Twitter. We have seen beautifully crafted advertising designs of some famous footballers doting on a can of soft drink on YouTube, and a TV program where a brand of alcohol was repetitively used. We have a plethora of examples of where the media has supported the unhealthy food industry. It is a source of worry because the media is everywhere. Everywhere you turn; there is a chance of seeing an ad that promotes a meal that is unhealthy. We are being coaxed and edged on, with sophisticated persuasion, to buy foods that will ultimately be dangerous to our health. Companies are employing specialists and scientists to engineer their products into being more habit-forming. They are making their products so irresistible that we're left licking our fingers and going back for more. Food corporations are deploying cutting-edge technology, such as the type of brain imaging technique that is deployed in the cure of addiction. Only in their case, they put subjects in machines and feed them one of those unhealthy and habit-forming foods to study how much they can tweak the ingredients in the foods to be more habit-forming.

Sugar is one ingredient they've deployed expertly in this regard. You'll be shocked to find out that 74% of foods in your grocery store have sugar added to them, and they don't have to be sweet. This has brought about some catastrophic effects. Children are being diagnosed with adult diseases. Type 2 diabetes that was known to affect only adults some years ago is gradually becoming common amongst children. The statistics are scary, as it shows that one out of every four American teenagers is either pre-diabetic or diabetic.

It doesn't end there. These days, diseases that didn't exist some 50 years ago are appearing now. Diagnosis of non-alcoholic fatty liver disease wasn't known until 1980. This disease is another condition that is linked to a poor diet or large consumption of sugar. According to Laura Schmidt, sugar scientist at the University of California, San Francisco's (UCSF) Professor of Health Policy, and this disease will be the leading cause of liver transplant in 2020. These and many more are the ills that the media is promoting in the name of marketing. They're after what an ad campaign will add to the purse and not what will happen to the person afterward, and as long as they're not breaking any known law, they will keep doing the same thing.

You must note that the media isn't your ally as you try to break away from eating unhealthy foods. It will try to knock you off your perch by continually putting up banners and videos of unhealthy foods in your face. You must have a strategy to counter everything that the media will do. You must be prepared to face them when you're trying to withdraw from the addiction you have. If you love pizza and want to quit eating it, be ready to be bombarded with images and videos about its taste. The following tips will help you.

Limit your exposure to media ads

The first and most obvious one is for you to limit the amount of exposure you have to media ads that promote these unhealthy habits on TV, radio, internet, and social media. Be selective of what you watch. You should consider sacrificing the show for your wellness; it would be a great motivation. On the internet, you can initiate the ad-blocker option on your browser—that way you'll block yourself from viewing ads of all kinds. Twitter has a feature that allows you to mute words you don't want to see on your feed. Get the buzzwords these companies use and block them accordingly. You can block all handles that bring anything close to an unhealthy diet to your timeline. When you limit your exposure to such ads, they will have less persuasive power over you.

See beyond the seductive marketing

You have to discipline yourself to see beyond the marketing gimmicks. Marketers want to sell and nothing more. The media will gladly help them do that. The most important question is if you'll allow some trendy two-minute video to determine your health status for the rest of your life. It's common for marketers and the media to use a celebrity who has a massive following in the digital space to sell a product. Again, are you going to allow someone who has been paid tens or hundreds or thousands of dollars for a video to promote a product he likely doesn't use to determine your health outlook? The answers depend on you alone. You should empower yourself with the ability to see beyond the lights.

The media has a massive reach. A simple idea in a small advertising company in New York might spread to a village in far Central Africa. Because of this, it is easy for the media to make something trendy in a matter of minutes. These trends influence people's behavior. Before hopping on a trend, especially one that has to do with food, do your research. Get the needed information and satisfy your curiosity. Don't just jump on it because others are jumping on it as well. Jump on it because it's good for your health.

Another point that supports this position is that our bodies are different. What worked for this person might not work for the next. Just because it is trending doesn't mean it is good, so be on the lookout.

Having information is one efficient way of dealing with everything the media comes at you with. Consult professionals. That way, you can protect yourself from any fallout that may come from following the media bandwagon.

Chapter 7

STOPPING THE UNHEALTHY DIET CRAZE

Our end goal is to mitigate or stop the consumption of sugar and an unhealthy diet. We need to eliminate deep and uncontrollable desires or cravings for unhealthy foods. Typically, foods that bring about cravings of these kinds are processed junk foods with very high levels of sugar. We know how dangerous sugar can be, and in fact, it is one of the worst things that can happen to your body. The sugars in some foods like vegetables and fruits have little or no harmful effects on the body because they are excellent sources of healthy vitamins and minerals. The problem lies with *added sugar* found in processed foods, which is a common feature in an unhealthy diet. Data from the National Cancer Institute's Epidemiology and Genomics Research Program showed that an average American consumes about 68 grams of sugar daily, more than the 25 grams for females and 37 grams for males recommended by experts. This goes to show how urgent it is to eliminate sugar, cravings for sugar, and other unhealthy diets from our lives.

First, we must reduce the volume of sugar-filled drinks we consume, a no-brainer on a keto diet. Most times, we turn the bottle on its head and empty the contents into our stomachs without knowing the content. A considerable number of our famous drinks have a significant percentage of added sugar. Data from the Center for Nutrition Policy and Promotion of the United States Department of Agriculture shows that energy drinks, sodas, fruit drinks, and sports drinks cumulatively make up 44% of the added sugar in a typical American diet. Smoothies and other healthy juices can also contain incredible amounts of sugar. If you are in the practice of always drinking something, consider changing your sugary drinks to either water (no calorie content), homemade soda (clean water with a squeeze of lime or fresh lemon), mixing water with cucumber and mint (an excellent combination especially when the weather is warm), fruit or herbal tea, or unsweetened tea.

Cutting away sugary drinks from your diet isn't only an "eat healthy" affair. It can go a long way in helping you maintain your weight at a healthy level.

It is not logical to cut sugary drinks and still hang on to sugary desserts. Most desserts don't add anything to the body in the form of nutritional values. Instead, they bring with their sweet taste an increase in your blood sugar levels and cause you to feel tired and hungry. They get you hooked to their sweetness to the point where you start to crave more. Desserts that are grain or dairy-based, like pies, cakes, ice cream, and doughnuts make up for more than 18% of added sugar intake in a typical American diet. Imagine the amount of sugar your body will be receiving if you go out for a picnic with friends and you consume two soft drinks and three doughnuts. If the taste is what pushes you to consume it, consider these mouthwatering keto delicacies that make up for all those cravings without knocking you out of ketosis:

- Keto brownies (made with sugar-free dark cocoa powder, xantham gum, and almond flour)
- Keto marshmallow treats (made with coconut, egg whites, gelatin, apple cider vinegar, and Himalayan salt)
- Keto chocolate cupcakes (made with coconut flour, cocoa powder, avocado oil, and full-fat coconut milk)
- Coconut cupcakes (made with cacao butter, coconut, and cinnamon)

Ketchup and other sauces are familiar sights in our kitchens. Many people aren't aware of the shocking sugar content it has. SELF Nutrition Data states that for every teaspoon of ketchup serving you take; you may be consuming 4 grams of sugar! To be sure, read the label to know what you're consuming. Try fresh or dried herbs or spices. They have neither calories nor sugar and can address tremendous benefits to the body. Vinegar, pesto, Harissa paste, and yellow mustard are options you can choose from.

One other point to note is how to defeat sugar cravings. We've learned in previous chapters that some of these foods are engineered to be habit-forming, with sugar as a key ingredient. To avoid sugar cravings, make sure you are eating the right amount of carb, protein, and fat ratio. Having more fats in your diet will help reduce those cravings.

Fats are slower to digest and ensure you are not having more proteins than necessary. The keto diet states that you must reduce your carbs, but it doesn't state that your protein intake should be heavily increased. The focus here is a large increment of your fat intake. On the standard keto diet, you must have 75 percent fat, 20 percent protein, and 5 percent carbohydrate.

Do you know that foods that are low in fat like yogurt, peanut butter, and salad dressing have more sugar and sometimes more calories than their full-fat counterpart? More sugar and more calories equal weight gain. A simple 13-gram small fat vanilla yogurt serving contains a whopping 16 grams of sugar and 96 calories! The same amount of full-fat plain yogurt contains only 5 grams of sugar and 69 calories! It is expedient that while you're trying to cut back on unhealthy foods, go for the full-fat version. They will make you healthier and help you to watch your weight.

Eat whole and fresh foods.

Eat more of meals that have not undergone any form of processing and have no additives or any other artificial workings. The exact opposite of whole foods is ultra-processed foods. They are foods that have sugar, salt, Trans fats, and other ingredients that are usually not used while cooking at home. They're made up of colors, artificial flavors, and other fake niceties. Desserts, cereals, pies, pizzas, and soft drinks are good examples of ultra-processed foods. Ultra-processed foods are not the same as conventional processed foods. In traditional processed foods, minimal ingredients are added, most of which you'll find in a typical kitchen. Examples of such kinds of foods are bread and cheese. This work states that 90% of added sugar in an average American diet is from ultra-processed foods, while only 8.7% is from food made at home. Surprisingly, junk foods aren't the only source. Seemingly healthy foods like canned pasta sauce can be a huge source of sugar, having it in alarming amounts.

You could say that the essence of eating healthy is to eat whole foods. Try as much as possible to make your foods at home. If you're not a good cook, there are lots of materials online that you can learn from, and you don't need to cook elaborate meals. Try simple options like marinating fish or meats in herbs, any way you prefer it, with spices and olive oil, and you'll get something delicious.

Avoid having canned foods. It was harder to control the carb contents when eating from the can. Make sure you stick with freshly prepared meals, so you won't eat more carbs because the labels didn't point them out.

While you try to replace foods that aren't healthy, you should not accept everything that comes your way just because "healthy" is written on it.

For example, John always eats candy bars. After reading online materials about how damaging they can be to his health, he decides to stop eating them and search for a healthy alternative. What he might not know is that such options might contain the same amount of sugar, if not more, than what he is avoiding. Some granola bars can contain as much as 32 grams of sugar. Whatever alternatives you settle for, make sure that you're not moving from the pot into the fire. A handful of nuts are a good source of calories and protein.

Even when you have to buy canned products lie tuna and seafood, reading labels should occupy a spot in the list where you outline what you should do while shopping. Look for hidden ingredients. Many packed soups might also contain high sodium which doesn't even point out that you are getting enough protein. When you have too high sodium in your diet without filling protein, it can promote sugar cravings.

Cutting away sugar consumption isn't as easy as stopping eating any food that tastes sugary. Some foods, though lacking a sweet taste, are high in sugar content. Food corporations know that you'll be on the lookout for sugar. Some familiar names you should be on the lookout for are cane sugar, rice syrup, molasses, maltose, invert sugar, dextrose, etc. In the US, it is becoming easier to identify goods with added sugar. The US Food and Drug Administration (FDA) has made alterations to its rules so that companies are compelled to disclose the number of added sugars on the list of ingredients used to make a product in grams and to add percentages of the amount to be taken daily.

Consider natural sweeteners, such as stevia. Stevia is produced from the leaves of a plant called *stevia rebaudiana.* This plant has no calorie content. Erythritol is another good example of a natural sweetener. It is found in fruits. Xylitol is another natural sweetener that is found in many fruits and vegetables.

Cut that unhealthy diet away! Stop the sugar! Start eating healthy!

Aside from looking out for sugar in your canned vegetables and soups, remember that canned foods undergo heating at the time of production to kill off bacteria. Therefore, your canned foods are not good sources of vitamins, antioxidants, and some minerals. A lot of canned foods, especially canned soups are also loaded with MSGs, so read your labels carefully. You should even understand that your canned foods have higher glycemic index than usually proclaimed by the company. This is not a deliberate act but arises because those canned foods are usually heated to kill bacteria which accelerate the glycemic index as well. So, you can make more of your sauces, soups, and vegetables than buying the canned variants.

So, the bottom line to avoid a lot of problems with canned foods:

- Avoid having them when you can
- Add additional servings of non-starchy vegetables
- Read labels for hidden ingredients.
- Consume more raw vegetables or make them slightly steamed

Tip: A word on cold pasteurization

Some food products are also created without heat. They are passed through ionizing radiation to alter those micro-organisms genetically and reduce the risks to illness. Cold pasteurization might look like a good thing right now, but the researches on this one is not enough. So, you are much better off sticking with freshly cooked meals.

Conclusion

We will always eat. If not to satisfy hunger, to satisfy a craving or to keep our gums busy. The world is replete with different types of food from various origins—a delight for foodies. A more fantastic reality is how you can eat foods from different continents in one day. The world has been sewn into a garment by the needle of technology.

Beginning a new weight loss diet is not always a simple transition, but you can achieve it, unstuck yourself from the mindset that you can't do and step up to your can-do attitude.

Avoiding a problematic situation is not a secret bonus to getting where you want to be. You still have all it takes to unlearn those habits you developed over the years. The keto and your persistence can get you what you always dreamed off. Everyone knows that challenges lead to growth. So, embrace this challenge. You have an embedded need to grow, learn, adjust, adapt and ascribe to become something better. So, do something about it!

To help you remember what you have learned in this guide, here's a recap:

- **Research and understand what it takes to do keto-** this includes understanding the basics of nutrition, calories, calorie reading, and looking out for hidden food ingredients that might disrupt your goal.
- **Get rid of unhealthy foods out of your home or office** – there is no fun in putting yourself through the confusion about whether you should go with a craving or not. Get them out, so they can stay out of mind.
- **Avoid the "all or nothing approach"** – There is no perfect way to start the keto plan. There is no ideal time or strategy. Begin today, plan a few days or week at a time and in the long run; your new habits will stick.
- **Focus on the process, not the outcome -** avoid setting a weight plan, focus on cultivating habits, so that long after you have transitioned into a more defined food plan, the habits of choosing healthy choices will stick.
- **Have a game plan every step of the way** – it's no use setting up a time table that only shows the three meals you will eat in a day, think about your work, family and

other responsibilities. Think about snack periods, desserts, midnight snacks, holidays, eat-outs, parties, conferences, and everything that would influence your diet plan.

- **Get a list of what motivates you** – understand what you truly want at the end of the day, write them down and make that list handy. You will be happy you did so on those days when you can't remember your motivations.

- **Get an accountability partner** – As humans, we are wired to connect, interact, and commit to each other. Get someone in your life to be the ear you would run to when things aren't going too well. That person can serve as your partner in this fight or the person that can remind you how strong you are when you forget.

You have what it takes to become better in every way. Don't try so hard; go with the flow. Give yourself breaks from time to time. Review your progress and adapt accordingly. Celebrate each milestone you conquer. And in the end, always remember that every step you take to become what you want, to shed off that weight, to live healthier and to enjoy your life to the fullest, is so worth it. Take that step, and the rest will fall into place.

www.ingramcontent.com/pod-product-compliance
Lightning Source LLC
Chambersburg PA
CBHW081604250726
48653CB00009B/3558